The Cav

Your Guide to a Paleo Lifestyle

Eating Healthy Doesn't Have to be Hard!

BY: Nancy Silverman

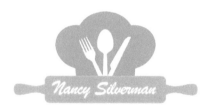

COPYRIGHT NOTICES

My Heartfelt Thanks and A Special Reward for Your Purchase!

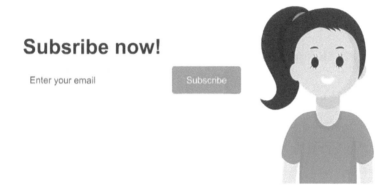

https://nancy.gr8.com

My heartfelt thanks at purchasing my book and I hope you enjoy it! As a special bonus, you will now be eligible to receive books absolutely free on a weekly basis! Get started by entering your email address in the box above to subscribe. A notification will be emailed to you of my free promotions, no purchase necessary! With little effort, you will be eligible for free and discounted books daily. In addition to this amazing gift, a reminder will be sent 1-2 days before the offer expires to remind you not to miss out. Enter now to start enjoying this special offer!

Table of Contents

Chapter 1 – 6 Paleo Appetizers and Snacks 7

    (1)   Lemon Chicken with Herbs 8

    (2)   Roasted Brittle Sprouts........................... 10

    (3)   Irish Cabbage and Bacon......................... 12

    (4)   Garlic Cauliflower 14

    (5)   Vegetable Medley................................... 16

    (6)   Paleo Walnut Squash 18

Chapter 2 – 6 Paleo Breakfast Recipes 19

    (1)   Paleo Pancakes 20

    (2)   Eggs and Zucchini 22

    (3)   Jalapeno-Bacon Egg in Cups 23

    (4)   Vegetable Casserole................................ 25

    (5)   Poached Eggs 27

    (6)   Zucchini and Ham Loaf.......................... 29

Chapter 3 – 6 Healthy Lunch Recipes to Reduce Weight 31

    (1)   Mushroom Salad 32

    (2)   Tuna and Avocado Cups 34

    (3)   Delicious Paleo Bread 36

    (4)   Chicken and Avocado Salad 38

    (5)   Chicken Salad with Vinegar 40

    (6)   Avocado and Egg Salad 42

Chapter 4 – 6 Paleo Dinner Recipes for Weight Loss 43

    (1)   Stuffed Peppers and Vegetables 44

    (2)   Stuffed Chicken 46

    (3)   Pork Roast with Rosemary 49

    (4)   Orange Seared Salmon 51

    (5)   Paleo Salmon with Pecan-Maple 53

    (6)   Cauliflower Chowder 55

Chapter 5 – 6 Paleo Dessert Recipes 57

    (1)   Paleo Butter Cookies 58

(2)   Raspberry Pop Slices 60

(3)   Chocolate Muffins 62

(4)   Pumpkin Cookies.................................. 64

(5)   Date and Coconut Bars.......................... 66

(6)   Strawberry Cookies............................... 68

About the Author.................................... 70

Author's Afterthoughts......................... 72

Chapter 1 – 6 Paleo Appetizers and Snacks

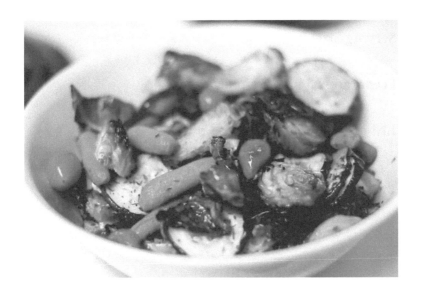

There are some delicious snacks and appetizers that you can enjoy with your paleo diet. These are healthy and easy to cook.

(1) Lemon Chicken with Herbs

It is a delicious and simple dish to cook your favorite lemon chicken with herbs. You can serve it with special spices.

Serving Size: 2

Preparation Time: 25 minutes

List of Ingredients:

- Olive oil: 1 Tbsp.
- Chicken (boneless and skinless): 2 breasts (halves)
- Lemon: 1
- Dried oregano: 1 pinch
- Fresh parsley: 2 sprigs for garnishing
- Pepper and salt: as per taste

||||||||||||||||||||||||||||||||||||||||||||||||||||||||||||||

Instructions:

Cut lemon and squeeze juice of only ½ lemon on chicken. Sprinkle salt as per taste and keep it aside for almost 10 minutes.

Heat oil in one skillet over medium heat and put the chicken in hot oil to sauté. Squeeze juice of remaining lemon and season with oregano and pepper as per taste. Sauté each side of chicken for almost 5 – 10 minutes, until juices dry. Garnish with parsley and serve.

(2) Roasted Brittle Sprouts

You can serve delicious brittle sprouts with salty and sweet sauce as per your taste. This recipe is easy and simple.

Serving Size: 6

Preparation Time: 1 hour

List of Ingredients:

- Brussels sprouts (trim ends and remove yellow leaves): 1 ½ pounds
- Kosher salt: 1 tsp.
- Olive oil: 3
- Black pepper (ground): ½ tsp.

|||||||||||||||||||||||||||||||||||||||||||||||||||||||||

Instructions:

Preheat your oven to almost 400 °F.

Put trimmed Brussels, pepper, salt and olive oil in one resealable plastic bag. Seal this bag tightly and shake well to coat Brussels. Pour Brussels on your baking sheet and put on the center of your oven rack.

Roast in your preheated oven for almost 30 – 45 minutes. Shake pan after every 5 – 7 minutes to make them equally brown. Reduce heat to avoid burning. Let them dark brown and adjust seasoning as per taste. Serve immediately.

(3) Irish Cabbage and Bacon

If you want to serve delicious cabbage with bacon, follow this delicious method and fill your stomach.

Serving Size: 6

Preparation Time: 25 minutes

List of Ingredients:

- Cabbage (cored and chopped): 1 head
- Bacon: 12ounces
- Bacon drippings: ¼ cup
- Black pepper (ground): as per taste

||||||||||||||||||||||||||||||||||||||||||||||||||||||||||||||

Instructions:

Cook bacon in your deep skillet on medium heat to make them crispy. It will take 5 – 7 minutes. Drain bacon on one plate lined with paper towel. Reserve almost ¼ cup bacon drippings in the skillet.

Cook cabbage in bacon dripping on medium flame to wilt cabbage. It will take almost 5 – 7 minutes. Crumble bacon on cabbage, stir well and cook for 2 – 3 minutes again. Sprinkle some black pepper and serve.

(4) Garlic Cauliflower

Your family will surely like this recipe because of its unique taste and beautiful colors.

Serving Size: 6

Preparation Time: 40 minutes

List of Ingredients:

- Minced garlic: 2 Tbsp.
- Parmesan cheese (grated): 1/3 cup
- Black Pepper (ground) and salt: as per taste
- Olive oil: 3 Tbsp.
- Chopped parsley: 1 Tbsp.
- Cauliflower (florets): 1 large head

|||||||||||||||||||||||||||||||||||||||||||||||||||||||||||||||

Instructions:

Preheat your oven to almost 450 °F. Grease one casserole dish.

Put garlic and olive oil in one resealable bag and add cauliflower in this bag. Seal this bag and mix well to coat cauliflower florets. Pour in your greased casserole dish and sprinkle with pepper and salt as per taste.

Bake for almost 25 minutes, stir halfway and top with parmesan cheese. Broil for almost 3 – 5 minutes to make them golden brown. Serve hot.

(5) Vegetable Medley

You can make this savory and sweet colorful dish to serve as a side dish or salad. It is a light meal for your unwanted hunger.

Serving Size: 6

Preparation Time: 1 hour 55 minutes

List of Ingredients:

- Olive oil (divided): 2 Tbsp.
- Red peppers (roasted): ½ cup (1-inch pieces)
- Yam (peeled and chopped): 1 large
- Minced garlic: 2 cloves
- Parsnip (peeled and chopped): 1 large
- Chopped basil: ¼ cup
- Kosher salt: ½ tsp.
- Baby carrots: 1 cup
- Black pepper (ground): ½ tsp.
- Chopped Zucchini (i-inch slices): 1
- Trimmed and chopped asparagus (1-inch pieces): 1 bunch

Instructions:

Preheat your oven to almost 425 °F. Grease two baking sheets with one Tbsp. olive oil.

Put carrots, parsnips and yams on your baking sheets. Bake in your preheated oven for almost 30 minutes and add asparagus and zucchini. Drizzle with remaining olive oil and continue baking for approximately 30 minutes again. Once tender, take out vegetables from oven and let them cool on baking sheet for almost 30 minutes.

Toss roasted pepper with salt, pepper, basil and garlic in one large bowl to combine everything. Add roasted vegetables, toss them well to mix and serve at your room temperature.

(6) Paleo Walnut Squash

You can prepare this mouthwatering dish to serve over brown rice and pasta. It will be a good side dish for paleo diet.

Serving Size: 2

Preparation Time: 15 minutes

List of Ingredients:

- Coconut oil: 2 Tbsp.
- Walnuts: 1 cup
- Shredded yellow squash: 1 large
- Garlic minced: 3 cloves
- Tomato (large chunks): 1 large

||||||||||||||||||||||||||||||||||||||||||||||||||||||||||||||

Instructions:

Put the skillet over medium heat and melt coconut oil in this skillet. Stir in garlic, walnuts, tomato and squash. Cook for almost 5 minutes and stir frequently. Serve hot.

Chapter 2 – 6 Paleo Breakfast Recipes

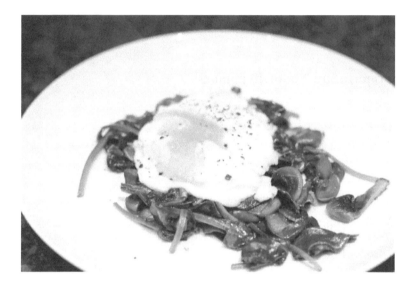

Start your day with a healthy and delicious breakfast. There are some delicious recipes to replace unhealthy breakfast with a healthy recipe:

(1) Paleo Pancakes

These classic pancakes are delicious for your breakfast. You can add agave nectar to make them sweet.

Serving Size: 2

Preparation Time: 40 minutes

List of Ingredients:

- Chicken or bacon slices: 3
- Coconut flour: 2 Tbsp.
- Baking soda: 1 pinch
- Eggs: 2
- Baking powder: 1 pinch
- Chopped banana: 1
- Salt: 1 pinch
- Vanilla extract: 1 tsp.
- Olive oil: as per your need

||||||||||||||||||||||||||||||||||||||||||||||||||||||

Instructions:

Grease one skillet and cook chicken slices over medium flame. Turn occasional to make them equally brown, and it may take almost 10 minutes. Drain chicken slices on some paper towels and crumble them.

Whisk banana and eggs in one bowl with one electric mixer to make it smooth and foamy. Stir in crumbled bacon pieces and vanilla extracts. Whisk salt, baking powder, baking soda, and coconut flour in egg mixture. Mix them well to combine everything. Leave the batter for almost 2 to 5 minutes.

Heat one griddle over medium flame and grease with olive oil. Drop two large spoonfuls of batter onto griddle and cook until bubbles appear on the top surface. It may take almost 3 – 4 minutes. Gently flip and cook another side for approximately 2 – 3 minutes. Replicate this procedure with remaining batter and serve hot pancakes.

Note: If you want to use bacon, there is no need to add olive oil. You can use bacon drippings.

(2) Eggs and Zucchini

You can serve zucchini and eggs in the breakfast. This delicious breakfast is easy to cook in the morning.

Serving Size: 1

Preparation Time: 10 minutes

List of Ingredients:

- Beaten egg: 1
- Olive oil: 2 tsp.
- Pepper and salt: as per taste
- Zucchini (sliced): 1 small

||||||||||||||||||||||||||||||||||||||||||||||||||||||||||||||||||

Instructions:

Heat oil in your small skillet over medium flame. Pour some oil and sauté zucchini slices until tender. Spread out all zucchini slices in one layer and pour whisked eggs over this layer. Cook for 3 to 4 minutes from both sides to make egg firm. Sprinkle pepper and salt as per taste and serve hot.

(3) Jalapeno-Bacon Egg in Cups

You can serve these classic eggs in breakfast. These are easy to carry with you in the office.

Serving Size: 4

Preparation Time: 40 minutes

List of Ingredients:

- Large eggs: 10
- Bacon slices (half cooked): 12
- Jalapeno peppers (sliced and seeded): 4
- Diced onion: ½
- Almond or coconut milk: ¼ cup
- Chopped bell pepper: ½ cup
- Garlic powder: ½ tsp.
- Black pepper (ground) and salt: as per taste

IIIIIIIIIIIIIIIIIIIIIIIIIIIIIIIIIIIIIIIIIIIIIIIIIIIIIIIIIIIII

Instructions:

Preheat your oven to almost 375 °F.

Take one bowl and whisk garlic powder, coconut milk, and eggs in this bowl. Season with pepper and salt as per taste and whisk these ingredients well.

Grease your muffin tins and line each cup with one bacon slice. Fill every hole with the whisked egg mixture, top with jalapeno, bell pepper, and diced onion.

Put this muffin tin in your preheated oven and bake for almost 20 – 25 minutes. Serve hot.

(4) Vegetable Casserole

You can enjoy a healthy breakfast with healthy fat and protein. Feel free to add chicken or bacon to casserole.

Serving Size: 4

Preparation Time: 45 minutes

List of Ingredients:

- Sweet potatoes or Russet (shredded): 2
- Diced onion: 1
- Minced garlic: 2 cloves
- Mushrooms (sliced): 1 cup
- Diced bell pepper: 1
- Fresh spinach: 1 cup
- Diced grape tomatoes: ½ cup
- Eggs: 12
- Olive oil: 1 to 2 Tbsp.
- Ground black pepper and salt: as per taste

IIIIIIIIIIIIIIIIIIIIIIIIIIIIIIIIIIIIIIIIIIIIIIIIIIIIII

Instructions:

Preheat your oven to almost 375 °F.

Pour olive oil in one skillet and add shredded russet and sauté on medium heat for almost 3 minutes.

Cover this skillet and cook for 3 minutes again over medium heat and put in one layer in the base of a greased baking dish.

Add olive oil to your skillet again and sauté garlic and onion for 3 minutes. Add sliced mushrooms and bell pepper, cook for 4 – 5 minutes. Mix in tomatoes and spinach during final 2 minutes.

Turn off heat and put vegetables on the top of shredded potatoes in your baking dish.

Take one large bowl and whisk eggs together. Sprinkle some pepper and salt as per taste. Pour egg mixture over the vegetable-filled baking dish and put it in the oven. Bake for 40 – 45 minutes and serve hot.

(5) Poached Eggs

You can flavor your poached eggs with bacon crumbles, herbs and tomatoes. It will be a good breakfast.

Serving Size: 4

Preparation Time: 40 minutes

List of Ingredients:

- Large eggs: 8
- Chopped garlic: 4 cloves
- Chicken stock: ¼ cup
- Minced onion: ½
- Crushed tomatoes: 2 cups
- Minced basil: 4 Tbsp.
- Minced parsley: 4 Tbsp.
- Olive oil: 2 Tbsp.
- Pre-cooked and crumble bacon: 4 – 6 slices
- Black pepper (ground) and sea salt: as per taste

Instructions:

Heat oil over medium flame in one skillet. Sauté onion and garlic in this skillet to make them soft.

Add basil and parsley in this skillet and cook for almost 1 minute. Stir frequently and pour crushed tomatoes, pepper, salt and chicken stock in this mixture. Let it boil and simmer for nearly 5 minutes.

Make 8 holes in this mixture and gently crack all eggs one by one in this sauce. Cover your skillet and let this mixture simmer for 10 - 12 minutes.

Top with crushed bacon and basil serve hot.

(6) Zucchini and Ham Loaf

You can make a delicious brunch during holidays with different vegetables and meat.

Serving Size: 4

Preparation Time: 45 minutes

List of Ingredients:

- Eggs: 10
- Zucchini (sliced): 2
- Minced garlic: 2 cloves
- Sliced onion: 1
- Ham (cubes): 1 cup
- Minced parsley: 1 Tbsp.
- Olive oil: as per your need
- Black pepper and salt: as per taste

IIIIIIIIIIIIIIIIIIIIIIIIIIIIIIIIIIIIIIIIIIIIIIIIIIIIIIIIIIIII

Instructions:

Heat olive oil in your skillet over medium flame and add sliced zucchini with pepper and salt. Mix them well and cook for almost 10 minutes. Add garlic and onion to cook for 10 minutes again. Put bell pepper and ham in this pan with sliced zucchini and cook for another 6 minutes.

Preheat your oven to almost 400 °F.

Line one loaf pan with baking or parchment paper.

Take one bowl and whisk parsley and eggs together. Sprinkle with some pepper and salt and whisk them well.

Put ham and zucchini mixture in the prepared loaf pan and pour eggs on the top of this mix. Put it in your preheated oven and cook for almost 20 – 25 minutes. Leave it for approximately 5 minutes before making slices and enjoy this delicious bread.

Chapter 3 – 6 Healthy Lunch Recipes to Reduce Weight

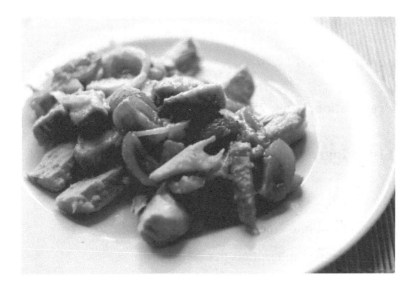

You should eat fresh and healthy in lunch to reduce weight and increase your strength. There are a few recipes to make your work easy. You can enjoy salads as your Paleo lunch.

(1) Mushroom Salad

You can enjoy this spicy mushroom salad with balsamic vinegar in lunch. This recipe is specially good for mushroom lovers.

Serving Size: 4

Preparation Time: 25 minutes

List of Ingredients:

- Olive oil: 1 Tbsp.
- Balsamic vinegar: 2 ½ Tbsp.
- Pepper and salt: as per taste
- Fresh mushrooms (sliced): 1 ½ cups
- Baby greens (mix): 10 ounces
- Chopped garlic: 1 clove (optional)
- Olive oil: 2 ½ Tbsp.

‖‖‖

Instructions:

Heat one Tbsp. oil in your skillet over medium heat and cook mushrooms in this oil until soft. Continue cooking until the juices of mushrooms have decreased to only two Tbsp..

Mix in remaining oil, salt, pepper and balsamic vinegar to blend everything. Turn off heat and leave the mushrooms in this pan to let them warm. You can't mix greens in hot mushrooms; otherwise, they will wilt excessively.

Put mix baby greens in your serving bowl and pour warm mushroom blend over them. Toss this mix and serve instantly.

(2) Tuna and Avocado Cups

Avocado has numerous benefits and you can mix it with tuna to increase advantages of this recipe.

Serving Size: 2

Preparation Time: 10 minutes

List of Ingredients:

- Tuna solid white in water (drained): 5 ounces
- Dry mustard: ¼ tsp.
- Minced celery: 2 Tbsp.
- Lemon pepper: 1/8 tsp.
- Minced onion: 2 Tbsp.
- Black pepper (ground) and Pink salt: as per taste
- Ripe avocado (halved and pitted): 1 large
- Fresh dill (minced): 2 Tbsp.
- Olive oil Mayo: 2 Tbsp.
- Celery salt: ¼ tsp.
- Lemon wedges: only for serving

||||||||||||||||||||||||||||||||||||||||||||||||||||||||

Instructions:

Take one bowl and slowly mix tuna, black pepper, lemon pepper, mustard, salt, mayo, dill, onion, and salary in this bowl. Mix them well and stuff the avocado halves with tuna mixture. Serve instantly with some lemon wedges.

(3) Delicious Paleo Bread

You can serve this delicious bread in breakfast or lunch with salads. This will be a healthy way to fill your stomach.

Serving Size: 8

Preparation Time: 1 hour 25 minutes

List of Ingredients:

- Almond flour: 1 ½ cups
- Pumpkin puree: 15 ounces
- Large eggs: 4
- Coconut flour: ½ cup
- Maple syrup: ½ cup
- Pumpkin pie seasoning/spice: 5 tsp.
- Coconut oil (melted): 5 Tbsp.
- Baking soda: 1 ½ tsp.
- Vanilla extract (pure): 2 tsp.
- Baking powder: 1 ½ tsp.
- Kosher salt: 1 tsp.

||||||||||||||||||||||||||||||||||||||||||||||||||||||||||||

Instructions:

Preheat your oven to almost 350 °F. Line one loaf pan (9x5-inch) with a parchment paper. Grease this paper with some coconut oil.

Take one bowl and mix salt, baking powder, baking soda, pumpkin spice, coconut flour and almond flour in this bowl. Mix these ingredients well.

Take another bowl and stir in vanilla extract, coconut oil, maple syrup, eggs, and pumpkin puree. Mix them well to make a smooth mixture. Add this wet mixture to your flour mixture and stir gently to moist all dry ingredients. Pour this batter into your loaf pan.

Bake in your preheated oven for almost 55 – 70 minutes and check with a toothpick or cake tester. If the tester comes out clean, the bread is ready. Leave bread in pan for almost 20 minutes and transfer to your wire rack let it completely cool.

(4) Chicken and Avocado Salad

This salad takes only 30 minutes and it will be a healthy lunch for your body. You can protect yourself from numerous diseases.

Serving Size: 4

Preparation Time: 20 minutes

List of Ingredients:

- Chopped chicken (cooked): 4 cups
- Raisins: ¼ cup
- Ripe avocadoes (peeled, pitted & mashed): 2
- Lime juice: 1 lime
- Chopped walnuts: ¼ cup
- Fresh basil (chopped): 2 Tbsp.
- Lettuce heads (leaves separated): 2
- Garlic salt: ½ tsp.
- Black pepper (ground): ½ tsp.

||||||||||||||||||||||||||||||||||||||||||||||||||||||||||||

Instructions:

Take one bowl and mix lime juice, avocados, salt, pepper and basil together in this bowl. Add walnuts, raisins, and chicken to this avocado mixture and mix them well. Divide mixtures into separate lettuce leaves and roll these leaves around filling. Serve!

(5) Chicken Salad with Vinegar

It will be a delicious and tangy salad with chicken and peppers. You can flavor this salad with apple and nuts.

Serving Size: 6

Preparation Time: 15 minutes

List of Ingredients:

- Cooked chicken (diced): 3 cups
- Chopped walnuts: ½ cup
- Diced apple: 1 cup
- Balsamic vinegar: 3 Tbsp.
- Olive oil: 5 Tbsp.
- Diced celery: ½ cup
- Pepper and salt: as per taste
- Chopped onions (green): 2

IIIIIIIIIIIIIIIIIIIIIIIIIIIIIIIIIIIIIIIIIIIIIIIIIIIIIIIIIIIII

Instructions:

Take one large bowl and toss celery, onion, walnuts, apple, and chicken in this bowl. Keep it aside.

Take one small bowl and whisk oil and vinegar together in this bowl. Pour this dressing over chicken mixture and sprinkle some pepper and salt. Mix all ingredients well and leave for almost 15 minutes. Mix again and serve.

(6) Avocado and Egg Salad

You can use avocado instead of adding mayo and serve in crackers or sandwich. It will be a healthy lunch.

Serving Size: 2

Preparation Time: 10 minutes

List of Ingredients:

- Mashed avocado (peeled and pitted): 1
- Chopped onion: 1 Tbsp.
- Chopped celery: 1 Tbsp.
- Chopped hard-boiled eggs (peeled): 3
- Salt: as per taste
- Pickle relish (Sweet): 1 Tbsp.

||||||||||||||||||||||||||||||||||||||||||||||||||||||||||||||||

Instructions:

Take one bowl and mix eggs and avocado together. Stir in salt, celery, onion and relish. Mix them well and serve with crackers or paleo bread.

Chapter 4 – 6 Paleo Dinner Recipes for Weight Loss

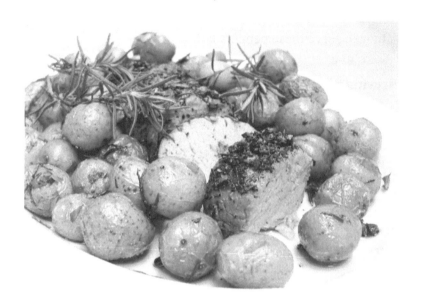

Your delicious paleo dinner will take a few minutes to prepare. There are some healthy and delicious methods to cook your favorite meals for dinner.

(1) Stuffed Peppers and Vegetables

Prepare delicious stuffed pepper with turkey and vegetables. You can serve these peppers hot.

Serving Size: 4

Preparation Time: 50 minutes

List of Ingredients:

- Bell pepper (green): 4 (remove tops and seeds)
- Belle pepper (yellow and chopped): ½
- Spinach (fresh): 1 cup
- Ground turkey: 1 pound
- Diced tomatoes: 14.5 ounces
- Olive oil: 2 Tbsp.
- Tomato paste: 1 Tbsp.
- Chopped onion: ½
- Italian seasoning: as per taste
- Mushrooms (sliced): 1 cup
- Garlic powder: as per taste
- Chopped zucchini: 1

- Pepper and salt: as per taste
- Bell pepper (red and chopped): 1/2

||||||||||||||||||||||||||||||||||||||||||||||||||||||||

Instructions:

Preheat your oven to almost 350 °F.

Wrap your bell peppers (green) in one aluminum foil and place in your baking dish. Bake bell peppers for approximately 15 minutes in your preheated oven. Take out from the oven.

In one skillet on medium flame, cook turkey and make it equally brown. Keep it aside.

Heat oil in this skillet and cook spinach, onion, bell pepper (red and yellow), zucchini and mushrooms in this skillet to tender vegetables. Return browned turkey to skillet and mix in tomatoes and tomato paste. Season with salt, pepper, garlic powder and delicious Italian seasoning as per taste.

Stuff all peppers (green) with this mixture and put peppers in your oven again to cook for almost 15 minutes.

(2) Stuffed Chicken

You can serve delicious chicken with guacamole and boost flavors of the chicken. This recipe will be good for special treats.

Serving Size: 4

Preparation Time: 1 hour

List of Ingredients:

- Chicken (skinless and boneless): 4 breasts
- Avocados (pitted and peeled): 2 ripe
- Diced onion (red): ¼ cup
- Diced tomato: ¼ cup
- Lime juice: 1 Tbsp.
- Minced garlic: 1 clove
- Chili powder: ¼ tsp.
- Ground cumin: ¼ tsp.
- Black pepper (ground) and sea salt: as per taste

Seasoned Flour List of Ingredients:

- Egg (lightly whisked): 1
- Almond flour: 1 cup
- Paprika: 1 Tbsp.
- Garlic powder: 1 tsp.
- Oregano (dried): 1 tsp.
- Chili powder: 1 tsp.
- Black pepper (ground) and salt: as per taste

||||||||||||||||||||||||||||||||||||||||||||||||||||||

Instructions:

Preheat your oven to almost 400 °F.

Pound every chicken breast to make it flat and thin with a rolling pin or meat mallet. Keep it aside.

Put avocados in one bowl and mash with a fork or potato masher. Add cumin, chili powder, lime juice, garlic, onion, and tomato in mashed avocados. Season this mixture as per taste and mix them well to combine everything. Guacamole is ready.

Spread an equal amount of guacamole in one thin layer over every flat chicken breast. Roll up every breast and use cooking string or toothpick to secure each breast. Keep it aside.

Take one bowl and mix pepper, salt, chili powder, oregano, garlic, paprika, and almond flour in this bowl. Carefully dredge every chicken breast in whisked egg and coat with your almond flour mix.

Put chicken in one greased baking dish and bake for almost 35 – 40 minutes. Check chicken for doneness and serve hot.

(3) Pork Roast with Rosemary

This pork roast with almonds and vinegar will be a good dinner for your Paleo diet. Serve this hot.

Serving Size: 6

Preparation Time: 2 hours 20 minutes

List of Ingredients:

- Pork tenderloin: 3 pounds
- Minced garlic: 2 cloves
- Olive oil: 1 Tbsp.
- Dried rosemary: 3 Tbsp.

||||||||||||||||||||||||||||||||||||||||||||||||||||||||

Instructions:

Preheat your oven to almost 375 °F.

Rub the tenderloin or roast liberally with your olive oil and spread garlic on it. Put it in your roasting pan (10x15-inch) and sprinkle some rosemary.

Bake it in your preheated oven for almost 2 hours or until the internal temperature of pork reaches approximately 145 °F. Serve hot!

(4) Orange Seared Salmon

Salmon is healthy for your paleo dinner and you can serve them with orange slices and fresh herbs.

Serving Size: 4

Preparation Time: 35 minutes

List of Ingredients:

- Salmon fillet without skin: 4
- Minced garlic: 2 cloves
- Minced rosemary: 2 tsp.
- Orange juice (fresh): 1 cup
- Lemon juice (fresh): 2 Tbsp.
- Chicken stock: ½ cup
- Orange zest: 2 tsp.
- Tapioca starch: 1 tsp.
- Olive oil: as per your need
- Black pepper (ground) and sea salt: as per taste

||||||||||||||||||||||||||||||||||||||||||||||||||||||

Instructions:

Season both sides of your salmon fillets and keep them aside.

Pour some olive oil in one skillet and put on medium heat. Cook these fillets in the skillet for almost 5 minutes for each side and keep them aside.

Take one bowl and combine orange zest, chicken stock, lemon juice and orange juice in this bowl. Use a similar skillet and cook rosemary and garlic for almost 2 minutes. Pour the mixture of orange juice in skillet and let it boil.

Reduce flame to medium-low and season as per your taste. If you want a thick sauce, you can mix tapioca starch and cold water (1 Tbsp.) and add it to your skillet.

Return salmon fillets to this skillet and spoon sauce over salmon fillets. Serve hot.

(5) Paleo Salmon with Pecan-Maple

This healthy and easy salmon is free from gluten and dairy. You can serve it with your favorite sauce.

Serving Size: 4

Preparation Time: 2 hours 27 minutes

List of Ingredients:

- Salmon: 4 ounces (4 fillets)
- Apple cider vinegar: 1 Tbsp.
- Smoked Paprika: 1 tsp.
- Black pepper (ground) and Salt: as per taste
- Pecans: ½ cup
- Chipotle ground pepper: ½ tsp.
- Onion powder: ½ tsp.
- Maple syrup (pure): 3 Tbsp.

||||||||||||||||||||||||||||||||||||||||||||||||||||||

Instructions:

Put some salmon fillets on one baking sheet and sprinkle with black pepper and salt. Keep it aside.

Combine onion powder, chipotle powder, paprika, vinegar, maple syrup and pecans in one blender or food processor. Pulse this blend to get a crumbly mixture. Spoon this mixture on the top of every salmon fillet, coat the top surface. Put this coated salmon for almost 2 – 3 hours in your fridge.

Preheat your oven to almost 425 °F. Bake salmon in your preheated oven for approximately 12 – 14 minutes, until the fish flakes with one fork.

(6) Cauliflower Chowder

You can make a delicious soup for dinner with some special flavors. You can serve hot chowder.

Serving Size: 4

Preparation Time: 45 minutes

List of Ingredients:

- Chopped cauliflower: 1 head
- Minced garlic: 2 cloves
- Diced onion: 1
- Chopped and peeled carrots: 2
- Diced celery: 2 stalks
- Chicken stock: 4 cups
- Coconut milk: 1 cup
- Ground cumin: 1 ¼ tsp.
- Ground turmeric: 1 tsp.
- Ground coriander: ½ tsp.
- Dill as per taste: optional
- Bacon slices (crumbled and cooked: 4
- Olive oil: as per taste
- Black pepper (ground) and salt: as per taste

Instructions:

Heat some olive oil in one saucepan over medium flame. Add celery, carrots, onion, and garlic to this pan and cook for almost 5 minutes.

Stir in chopped cauliflower and cook for almost 5 minutes. Stir occasionally and add coconut milk, coriander, turmeric, cumin and chicken stock in this pan. Let it boil and reduce heat to simmer this mixture for almost 15 minutes to tender vegetables. Sprinkle with some seasoning as per taste and garnish with fresh dill and bacon. Serve hot.

Chapter 5 – 6 Paleo Dessert Recipes

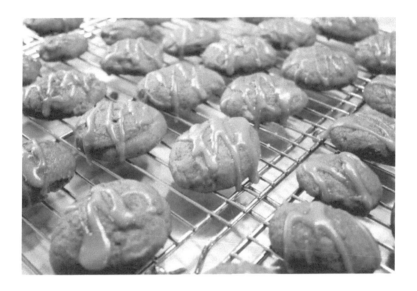

Paleo diet will not keep you away from your favorite sweet items. You can serve these delicious desserts that are healthy and easy to prepare.

(1) Paleo Butter Cookies

These delicious cookies are purely paleo and you can eat them without any fear of weight gain.

Serving Size: 8

Preparation Time: 30 minutes

List of Ingredients:

- Egg: 1
- Cashew butter: ½ cup
- Chopped dates (pitted): 2 Tbsp.
- Dried cranberries: ¼ cup
- Honey: 1 Tbsp.
- Chopped almonds: ¼ cup
- Coconut oil: 1 tsp.

|||||||||||||||||||||||||||||||||||||||||||||||||||||||||||||||

Instructions:

Preheat your oven to almost 350 °F.

Take one bowl and mix honey, dates, egg, coconut oil, almonds, cranberries and cashew butter in this bowl. Mix them well and put spoonfuls of this mixture on your nonstick baking dish/sheet with 1-inch distance.

Bake in your preheated oven for almost 12 minutes and let it cool for a few minutes to make them hard. You can secure them in one glass jar.

(2) Raspberry Pop Slices

You can enjoy the sweet taste of raspberries via these delicious pops. These are colorful and delicious popsicles.

Serving Size: 4

Preparation Time: 20 minutes

List of Ingredients:

- Raspberries (fresh): 1 ½ cups
- Water: 2 cups
- Tray of ice cubes
- Popsicle sticks (3 parallel pieces): 4 to 5

||||||||||||||||||||||||||||||||||||||||||||||||||||||||||

Instructions:

Combine raspberries and water in one saucepan over medium flame. Let it simmer for almost 10 – 15 minutes. Make sure the mixture should stick to one spoon.

Turn off heat and drain with the help of one fine sieve and remove unwanted seeds.

Pour this mixture into every hole of your ice cube tray.

Put one popsicle stick piece into every hole and freeze for almost 2 hours before eating. In case, the popsicle sticks are unable to stay upright in holes, stick ice tray in your freezer and freeze it for ½ hour and insert popsicle sticks.

You can add fresh pieces of raspberries to each popsicle before freezing them.

(3) Chocolate Muffins

There is no need to forget your love for chocolate because we have special bites for you.

Serving Size: 8

Preparation Time: 45 minutes

List of Ingredients:

- Ripe bananas (you can change fruit): 3
- Almond butter: 1 cup
- Cocoa powder: ½ cup
- Beaten egg: 1
- Vanilla extract: 2 tsp.
- Raw honey: 2 Tbsp.
- Muffin pan: mini

||||||||||||||||||||||||||||||||||||||||||||||||||||||||||

Instructions:

Preheat your oven to almost 375 °F.

Take one bowl and combine all ingredients. Mix them well to combine and fill every muffin tin with this mixture

Bake in your preheated oven for almost 25 – 30 minutes.

Let them cool in pan for almost 8 minutes and serve.

(4) Pumpkin Cookies

You should not miss this delicious and healthy treat for holiday season. These cookies are great to secure in your glass jar.

Serving Size: 4

Preparation Time: 30 minutes

List of Ingredients:

- Pumpkin puree: 1 ½ cup
- Applesauce: ¼ cup
- Coconut milk (full-fat): ¼ cup
- Vanilla: 1 tsp.
- Almond meal: 1 cup
- Coconut flour: ½ cup
- Pumpkin spice: ½ tsp.

|||||||||||||||||||||||||||||||||||||||||||||||||||||||||

Instructions:

Preheat your oven to almost 350 °F.

Take one bowl and combine vanilla, applesauce, coconut milk and pumpkin puree in this bowl. Mix these ingredients well.

Slowly add almond meal and coconut flour to this bowl and mix them well.

Prepare a baking sheet by lining it with parchment paper or grease it. Drop spoonfuls of cookie mixture and make them flat with a fork. Put this cookie sheet in your oven and bake for almost 20 – 25 minutes. Let them cool on a wire rack and secure in a sterile mason jar.

(5) Date and Coconut Bars

This paleo snack is healthy for your active lifestyle. You can enjoy these bars before or after a workout.

Serving Size: 4

Preparation Time: 40 minutes

List of Ingredients:

- Silvered almonds: 1/3 cup
- Cashews: ¼ cup
- Flaked coconut: ½ cup
- Coconut oil: 1 tsp.
- Pitted dates: 10

||||||||||||||||||||||||||||||||||||||||||||||||||||||||||||||

Instructions:

Take one food processor and blend coconut and almond in this processor. Add dates and pulse again to combine everything. It is time to add coconut oil and cashews. Pulse this mixture again to make it thick. Transfer it to one waxed paper and make squares of this blend. Fold sides of this waxed paper toward the top and put in the fridge for almost 30 minutes.

(6) Strawberry Cookies

You should try these delicious cookies, but you will need one food dehydrator to make these cookies.

Serving Size: 24

Preparation Time: 24 hours

List of Ingredients:

- Fresh strawberries: 2 cups
- Raisins: 1 cup
- Blanched almonds: 2 cups

|||||||||||||||||||||||||||||||||||||||||||||||||||||||||||||

Instructions:

Soak almonds for one night in water.

Soak raisins in boiling water for almost five minutes and drain. Dice strawberries and raisins.

Coarsely grind almonds (soaked) and add them to your strawberry and raisin mixture. Mix them well.

Drop spoonfuls of batter on the plastic tray of the dehydrator and dehydrate for almost 24 hours at 105 °F. Turn cookies after 8 - 12 hours or after noticing that the one side is dry enough.

About the Author

Nancy Silverman is an accomplished chef from Essex, Vermont. Armed with her degree in Nutrition and Food Sciences from the University of Vermont, Nancy has excelled at creating e-books that contain healthy and delicious meals that anyone can make and everyone can enjoy. She improved her cooking skills at the New England Culinary Institute in Montpelier Vermont and she has been working at perfecting her culinary style since graduation. She claims that her life's work is always a work in progress and she only hopes to be an inspiration to aspiring chefs everywhere.

Her greatest joy is cooking in her modern kitchen with her family and creating inspiring and delicious meals. She often says that she has perfected her signature dishes based on her family's critique of each and every one.

Nancy has her own catering company and has also been fortunate enough to be head chef at some of Vermont's most exclusive restaurants. When a friend suggested she share some of her outstanding signature dishes, she decided to add cookbook author to her repertoire of personal achievements. Being a technological savvy woman, she felt the e-book realm would be a better fit and soon she had her first cookbook available online. As of today, Nancy has sold over 1,000 e-books and has shared her culinary experiences and brilliant recipes with people from all over the world! She plans on expanding into self-help books and dietary cookbooks, so stayed tuned!

Author's Afterthoughts

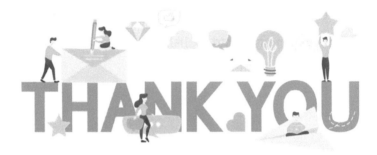

Thank you for making the decision to invest in one of my cookbooks! I cherish all my readers and hope you find joy in preparing these meals as I have.

There are so many books available and I am truly grateful that you decided to buy this one and follow it from beginning to end.

I love hearing from my readers on what they thought of this book and any value they received from reading it. As a personal favor, I would appreciate any feedback you can give in the form of a review on Amazon and please be honest! This kind of support will help others make an informed choice on and will help me tremendously in producing the best quality books possible.

My most heartfelt thanks,

Nancy Silverman

If you're interested in more of my books, be sure to follow my author page on Amazon (can be found on the link Bellow) or scan the QR-Code.

https://www.amazon.com/author/nancy-silverman

Made in United States
Troutdale, OR
06/27/2024

20850305R00051